Pressure Cooker

Recipes for Whole

Family

Easy, Delicious, Healthy Recipes For

Every Day!

Teresa M. Riley

Introduction

Considering the principle of diet in current times are based upon fasting, instead our keto instant pot is based upon the extreme decrease of carbs.

This kind of diet is based on the intake of specific foods that allow you to slim down faster permitting you to slim down approximately 3 kg each week.

You will certainly see how simple it will be to make these tasty meals with the tools available as well as you will certainly see that you will certainly be satisfied.

If you are reluctant concerning this fantastic diet plan you simply have to try it as well as analyze your results to a short time, trust me you will be pleased.

Bear in mind that the most effective method to reduce weight is to analyze your situation with the help of a specialist.

Healthy dishes

Turkey Tenderloin

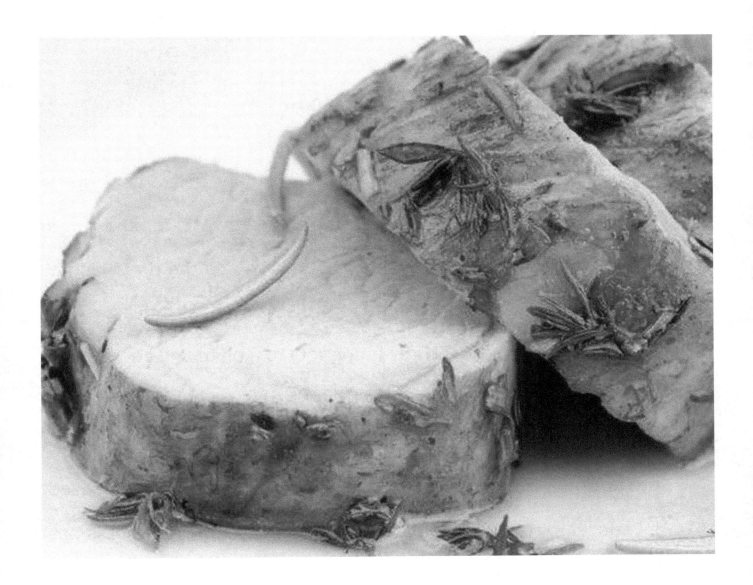

Ingredients for 4-6 servings:

1 Boneless Turkey Breast Tenderloin 4 T. Garlic Infused Oil 1 Medium Onion, cut into wedges 1 ½ c. Chicken Broth 1 t. Rosemary 1 t. Thyme 1. t. Oregano Salt and Pepper, to taste Cajun Rub, optional

Directions and total time – 30-60 m

• Turn Instant Pot on to sauté. Allow the inner pot to heat up. • Cover the turkey breast tenderloin with up to 2 T. oil and rub in the seasonings. • Once the inner pot is hot, add the remaining oil (2-3 T.) and turkey breast to the pot. Brown on all sides. • After browning, remove the turkey tenderloin to a plate and set aside. • Add 1 ½ c. of chicken broth to the pot. Use a wooden spatula to deglaze the bottom of the pot. Make sure all the browned bits on the bottom of the pot are scraped up. • Once the pot is deglazed, hit cancel. • Insert the trivet into the pot carefully (the pot is hot) and place the tenderloin on top of the trivet. Add in the onion wedges. • Place the lid on the pot and set the vent to sealing. •

Pressure cook on "High/Manual" for 30 minutes. • Once the turkey

is done cooking allow the pressure to release naturally.

Turkey with Drop Biscuit Dumplings

Ingredients for 8 servings:

Bones from a cooked bone-in turkey breast Trimmings from 1-2 leeks Trimmings from 3 carrots Trimmings from 3 celery stalks 1 teaspoon whole peppercorns 2 whole bay leaves 1 small sprig of fresh rosemary 5-6 sprigs of fresh thyme 2 whole garlic cloves 1 tablespoon apple cider vinegar Water For the stew: 1 teaspoon butter 2 teaspoons olive oil 1 ¼ cup small-diced carrots (about 3 medium carrots) 1 ¼ cup small-diced leeks (about 1 large or 2 small leeks) 1 ¼ cup small-diced celery (about 3 stalks) 1 teaspoon minced garlic 1 teaspoon finely chopped fresh thyme ½ teaspoon finely chopped fresh rosemary ¼ cup flour ½ cup white wine 5 cups turkey bone broth (from recipe above; or substitute with chicken or turkey stock) 4 cups shredded cooked turkey meat Salt and pepper to taste For the drop biscuits: 1 ¾ cups all-purpose flour (or 1 cup all-purpose and 1 cup white whole wheat) 2 teaspoons baking powder ½ teaspoon baking soda ½ teaspoon salt 4 tablespoons butter 1 cup cold low-fat buttermilk

Directions and total time – 1-2 h For the broth (optional):

• Place the bones of the turkey breast in the Instant Pot insert. Add the vegetable trimmings. Fill up to 1 inch below the max fill line with water. Add the peppercorns, bay leaves, fresh herbs, garlic, and cider vinegar. Place the lid on the Instant Pot and set to "sealing." Cook on high pressure for 45 minutes and allow for a 30-minute natural pressure release. • Carefully move the knob to "venting" and release any remainder of steam in the Instant Pot. Strain the broth through a fine-mesh strainer. Season to taste with salt. Cool completely before storing in the refrigerator. Remove 5 cups of broth for the dumpling stew. Chill the remainder and store in the fridge for when you reheat dumpling leftovers. For the stew: • Set the Instant Pot on "saute" mode. Add the butter and olive oil. Once the butter is melted, add the carrots, leeks, and celery. Saute until softened and translucent, about 5 minutes, being careful not to let anything burn on the bottom of the pot. Add the garlic, thyme, and rosemary, stirring until fragrant, about 30 seconds. Add the flour and stir to coat the vegetables. Add the wine to deglaze, scraping up any bits on the bottom and sides of the pot. Add the broth and shredded turkey, stirring until the mixture comes to a simmer, about 4 minutes. Press "cancel" on the Instant Pot to turn off the heat. Season to taste with salt and pepper. Remove the pot insert from the Instant Pot while you make the dumplings to ensure that nothing sticks to the bottom and the sides. • For the dumplings: • In a medium bowl, combine the flour, salt, baking powder, and baking soda. Melt the butter, and after cooling for 2-3 minutes, add it to the buttermilk. Let it stand in the buttermilk for 2-3 minutes. Stir the mixture together until the butter forms clumps in the buttermilk. Add this mixture to the flour mixture and use a rubber spatula to stir it into the flour until just combined. Use a small cookie dough scoop to scoop the drop biscuits into the turkey mixture in the Instant Pot insert. You should have 18-20 dumplings total. • Return the insert to the Instant Pot and place the lid on top. Set the knob to "sealing." Cook on high pressure for 3 minutes. Carefully quick release the pressure manually, allowing all the steam to escape. Ladle the stew and dumplings into bowls and serve warm! • Reheat leftovers and add extra turkey broth as needed to get the desired consistency you like as you reheat. • Note: if for some reason you get "burn" notice on the Instant Pot, no worries! Just release the pressure, remove the lid, and turn the Instant Pot to "saute" mode. Bring the mixture to a simmer and cook the dumplings, carefully stirring often with a rubber spatula, for 5 minutes. Ladle into bowls and serve. Stovetop instructions: • Place a large pot over medium heat. Add the butter and olive oil. Once the butter is melted, add the carrots, leeks, and celery. Saute for 5-6 minutes until softened and translucent. Add the garlic, thyme, and rosemary, stirring until fragrant, about 30 seconds. Add the flour and stir to coat the vegetables. Add the wine to deglaze, scraping up any bits on the bottom and sides of the pot. Add the broth and shredded turkey, stirring until the mixture comes to a simmer, about 4-5 minutes. • Use a small cookie dough scoop to scoop the drop biscuits into the turkey mixture. You should have 18-20 dumplings total. Place the lid on the pot and simmer over low heat for 10 minutes. Remove lid and serve

Apple Pie Granola

(Ready in about 1 hour 35 minutes | Servings 4)

Per serving: 234 Calories; 22.2g Fat; 9.5g Carbs; 2.5g Protein; 5.3g Sugars

Ingredients

3 tablespoons coconut oil 1 teaspoon stevia powder 1 cup coconut, shredded 1/4 cup walnuts, chopped 1 ½ tablespoons sunflower seeds 1 ½ tablespoons pumpkin seeds 1 teaspoon apple pie spice mix A pinch of salt 1 small apple, sliced

Directions Place coconut oil, stevia powder, coconut, walnuts, sunflower seeds, pumpkin seeds, apple pie spice mix, and salt in your Instant Pot. Secure the lid. Choose "Slow Cook" mode and High pressure; cook for 1 hours 30 minutes. Once cooking is complete, use a quick pressure release; carefully remove the lid.

Spoon into individual bowls, garnish with apples and serve warm.

Bon appétit!

Shirred Eggs with Peppers and Scallions

(Ready in about 10 minutes | Servings 4)

Per serving: 208 Calories; 18.7g Fat; 3.9g Carbs; 6.7g Protein; 2.3g Sugars

Ingredients

4 tablespoons butter, melted 4 tablespoons double cream 4 eggs 4 scallions, chopped 2 red peppers, seeded and chopped 1/2 teaspoon granulated garlic 1/4 teaspoon dill weed 1/4 teaspoon sea salt 1/4 teaspoon freshly ground pepper

Directions

Start by adding 1 cup of water and a metal rack to the Instant Pot. Grease the bottom and sides of each ramekin with melted butter. Divide the ingredients among the prepared four ramekins. Lower the ramekins onto the metal rack. Secure the lid. Choose "Manual" mode and High pressure; cook for 5 minutes. Once cooking is complete, use a natural pressure release; carefully remove the lid.

Bon appétit!

Hungarian Hot Pot

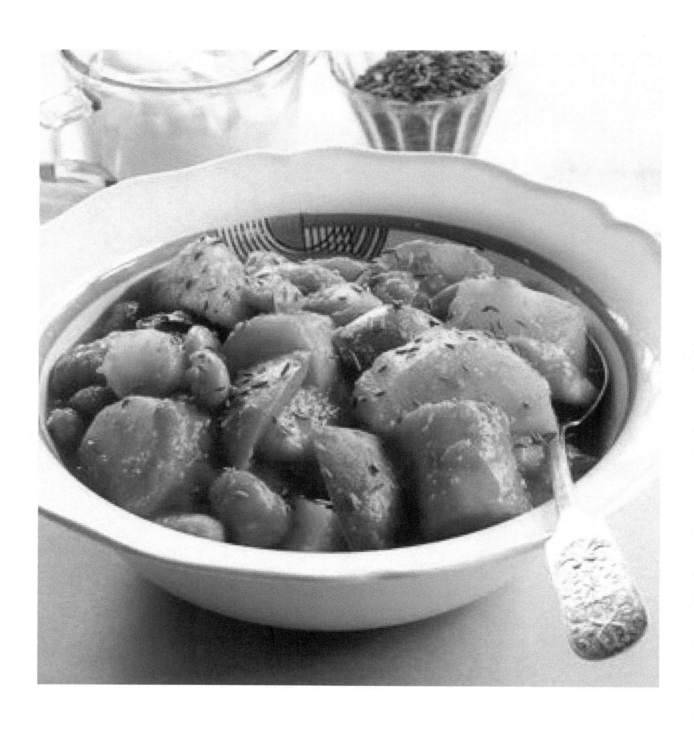

(Ready in about 15 minutes | Servings 4)

Per serving: 292 Calories; 21.6g Fat; 8.4g Carbs; 15.7g Protein; 3.5g Sugars

Ingredients

1 tablespoon grapeseed oil 9 ounces Hungarian smoked sausage, casing removed and sliced 1 carrot, cut into thick slices 1 celery stalk, diced 2 bell peppers, cut into wedges 2 cups roasted vegetable broth 1/2 cup shallot, peeled and diced Sea salt and ground black pepper, to taste 1/2 tablespoon hot pepper flakes 1 bay leaf 1/4 cup fresh cilantro leaves, roughly chopped

Directions

Press the "Sauté" button to heat up the Instant Pot. Now, heat the oil and brown the sausage for 2 to 3 minutes. Stir in the other ingredients. Secure the lid. Choose "Manual" mode and High pressure; cook for 10 minutes. Once cooking is complete, use a natural pressure release; carefully remove the lid. Bon appétit!

Dilled Cauliflower Purée with Au Jus Gravy

(Ready in about 20 minutes | Servings 4)

Per serving: 291 Calories; 26.6g Fat; 8.1g Carbs; 7.1g Protein; 4.5g Sugars

Ingredients

Cauliflower Purée: 1 head of fresh cauliflower, broken into florets 1/4 cup double cream 2 tablespoons butter 3 cloves garlic minced 4 tablespoons Romano cheese, grated 1 teaspoon dried dill weed Kosher salt and ground black pepper, to taste Gravy: 1 ½ cups beef stock 1/2 cup double cream 3 tablespoons butter

Directions

Add 1 cup of water and a steamer basket to the bottom of your Instant Pot. Then, arrange cauliflower in the steamer basket. Secure the lid. Choose "Manual" mode and Low pressure; cook for 3 minutes. Once cooking is complete, use a quick pressure release; carefully remove the lid. Now, puree the cauliflower with a potato masher. Add the remaining ingredients for the purée and stir well. Press the "Sauté" button to heat up the Instant Pot. Now, combine the ingredients for the gravy and let it simmer for 10 minutes. Stir until the gravy thickens down to a consistency of your liking. Serve cauliflower purée with the gravy on the side. Bon appétit!

Coconut Porridge with Berries

(Ready in about 10 minutes | Servings 2)

Per serving: 242 Calories; 20.7g Fat; 7.9g Carbs; 7.6g Protein; 2.8g Sugars

Ingredients

4 tablespoons coconut flour 1 tablespoon sunflower seeds 3 tablespoons flax meal 1 ¼ cups water 1/4 teaspoon coarse salt 1/4 teaspoon grated nutmeg 1/2 teaspoon ground cardamom 2 eggs, beaten 2 tablespoons coconut oil, softened 2 tablespoons Swerve 1/2 cup mixed berries, fresh or frozen (thawed)

Directions

Add all ingredients, except for mixed berries, to the Instant Pot. Secure the lid. Choose "Manual" mode and High pressure; cook for 5 minutes. Once cooking is complete, use a quick pressure release; carefully remove the lid. Divide between two bowls, top with berries, and serve hot. Bon appétit!

Zucchini Sloppy Joe's

(Ready in about 10 minutes | Servings 2

Per serving: 159 Calories; 9.8g Fat; 1.5g Carbs; 15.5g Protein; 0.7g Sugars

Ingredients

1 tablespoon olive oil 1/2 pound ground beef Salt and ground black pepper, to taste 1 medium-sized zucchini, cut into 4 slices lengthwise 1 tomato, sliced 4 lettuce leaves 2 teaspoons mustard

Directions

Add olive oil, ground beef, salt, and black pepper to your Instant Pot. Secure the lid. Choose "Manual" mode and High pressure; cook for 5 minutes. Once cooking is complete, use a natural pressure release; carefully remove the lid. Divide the ground meat mixture between 2 zucchini slices. Add tomato slices, lettuce, and mustard. Top with the second slice of zucchini. Bon appétit!

Fluffy Berry Cupcakes

(Ready in about 30 minutes | Servings 6)

Per serving: 238 Calories; 21.6g Fat; 4.1g Carbs; 7.5g Protein; 2.2g Sugars

Ingredients

1/4 cup coconut oil, softened 3 ounces cream cheese, softened 1/4 cup double cream 4 eggs 1/4 cup coconut flour 1/4 cup almond flour A pinch of salt 1/3 cup Swerve, granulated 1 teaspoon baking powder 1/4 teaspoon cardamom powder 1/2 teaspoon star anise, ground 1/2 cup fresh mixed berries

Directions

Start by adding 1 ½ cups of water and a metal rack to your Instant Pot. Mix coconut oil, cream cheese, and double cream in a bowl. Fold in the eggs, one at a time, and continue to mix until everything is well incorporated. In another bowl, thoroughly combine the flour, salt, Swerve, baking powder, cardamom, and anise. Add the cream/egg mixture to this dry mixture. Afterwards, fold in fresh berries and gently stir to combine. Divide the batter between silicone cupcake liners. Cover with a piece of foil. Place the cupcakes on the rack. Secure the lid. Choose "Manual" mode and High pressure; cook for 25 minutes. Once cooking is complete, use a natural pressure release; carefully remove the lid. Enjoy!

Salmon and Ricotta Fat Bombs

(Ready in about 15 minutes | Servings 6)

Per serving: 130 Calories; 9.1g Fat; 1.7g Carbs; 10.2g Protein; 0.5g Sugars

Ingredients

1/2 pound salmon fillets Salt and ground black pepper, to taste 1/4 teaspoon smoked paprika 1/4 teaspoon hot paprika 2 tablespoons butter, softened 4 ounces Ricotta cheese, room temperature 1/4 cup green onions, chopped 1 garlic clove, finely chopped 2 teaspoons fresh parsley, finely chopped

Directions

Start by adding 1 ½ cups of water and a metal rack to the bottom of your Instant Pot. Place the salmon on the metal rack. Secure the lid. Choose "Manual" mode and Low pressure; cook for 8 minutes. Once cooking is complete, use a quick pressure release;

carefully remove the lid. Chop the salmon. Add the salt, pepper, paprika, butter, cheese, onions, and garlic. Shape the mixture into balls and roll them in chopped parsley. Arrange fat bombs on a serving platter and enjoy!

Greek-Style Mushroom Muffins

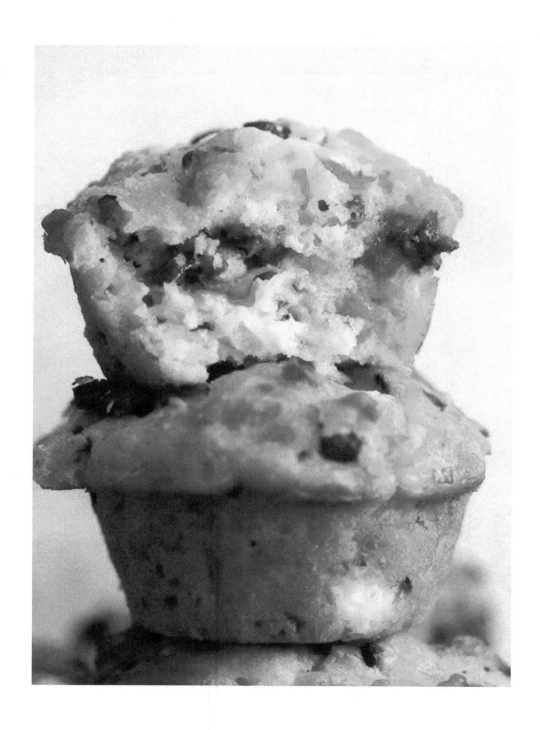

(Ready in about 10 minutes | Servings 6)

Per serving: 259 Calories; 18.9g Fat; 6.7g Carbs; 15.7g Protein; 3.9g Sugars

Ingredients

6 eggs 1 red onion, chopped 2 cups button mushrooms, chopped Sea salt and ground black pepper, to taste 1 ½ cups Feta cheese, shredded 1/2 cup Kalamata olives, pitted and sliced

Directions

Start by adding 1 ½ cups of water and a metal rack to the bottom of the Instant Pot. Spritz each muffin liner with a nonstick cooking spray. In a mixing bowl, thoroughly combine the eggs, onions, mushrooms, salt, and black pepper. Now, pour this mixture into the muffin liners. Secure the lid. Choose "Manual" mode and Low pressure; cook for 7 minutes. Once cooking is complete, use a quick pressure release; carefully remove the lid. Sprinkle cheese and olives on top of the cups; cover with the lid for a few minutes to allow it to melt. Enjoy!

Easy Spinach Dip

(Ready in about 5 minutes | Servings 10)

Per serving: 43 Calories; 1.7g Fat; 3.5g Carbs; 4.1g Protein; 1.3g Sugars

Ingredients

1 pound spinach 4 ounces Cottage cheese, at room temperature 4 ounces Cheddar cheese, grated 1 teaspoon garlic powder 1/2 teaspoon shallot powder 1/2 teaspoon celery seeds 1/2 teaspoon fennel seeds 1/2 teaspoon cayenne pepper Salt and black pepper, to taste

Directions

Add all of the above ingredients to your Instant Pot. Secure the lid. Choose "Manual" mode and High pressure; cook for 1 minute. Once cooking is complete, use a quick pressure release; carefully remove the lid. Serve warm or at room temperature. Bon appétit!

Cheesy Mustard Greens Dip

(Ready in about 10 minutes | Servings 10)

Per serving: 153 Calories; 10.6g Fat; 7g Carbs; 8.7g Protein; 3.6g Sugars

Ingredients

2 tablespoons butter, melted 20 ounces mustard greens 2 bell peppers, chopped 1 white onion, chopped 1 teaspoon garlic, minced Sea salt and ground black pepper, to taste 1 cup chicken stock 8 ounces Neufchâtel cheese, crumbled 1/2 teaspoon dried thyme 1/2 teaspoon dried dill 1/2 teaspoon turmeric powder 3/4 cup Romano cheese, preferably freshly grated

Directions

Add the butter, mustard greens, bell peppers, onion, and garlic to the Instant Pot. Secure the lid. Choose "Manual" mode and High pressure; cook for 3 minutes. Once cooking is complete, use a quick pressure release; carefully remove the lid. Then, add the remaining ingredients and press the "Sauté" button. Let it simmer until the cheese is melted; then, gently stir this mixture until everything is well incorporated. Serve with your favorite low-carb dippers.

Colorful Stuffed Mushrooms

(Ready in about 10 minutes | Servings 5)

Per serving: 151 Calories; 9.2g Fat; 6g Carbs; 11.9g Protein; 3.6g Sugars

Ingredients

1 tablespoon butter, softened 1 shallot, chopped 2 cloves garlic, minced 1 ½ cups Cottage cheese, at room temperature 1/2 cup Romano cheese, grated 1 red bell pepper, chopped 1 green bell pepper, chopped 1 jalapeno pepper, minced 1/2 teaspoon dried basil 1/2 teaspoon dried oregano 1/2 teaspoon dried rosemary 10 medium-sized button mushrooms, stems removed

Directions

Press the "Sauté" button to heat up your Instant Pot. Once hot, melt the butter and sauté the shallots until tender and translucent. Stir in the garlic and cook an additional 30 seconds or until aromatic. Now, add the remaining ingredients, except for the mushroom caps, and stir to combine well. Then, fill the mushroom caps with this mixture. Add 1 cup of water and a steamer basket to you Instant Pot. Arrange the stuffed mushrooms in the steamer basket. Secure the lid. Choose "Manual" mode and High pressure; cook for 5 minutes. Once cooking is complete, use a quick pressure release; carefully remove the lid. Arrange the stuffed mushroom on a serving platter and serve. Enjoy!

Herbed and Caramelized Mushrooms

(Ready in about 10 minutes | Servings 4)

Per serving: 91 Calories; 6.4g Fat; 5.5g Carbs; 5.2g Protein; 2.8g Sugars

Ingredients

2 tablespoons butter, melted 20 ounces button mushrooms, brushed clean 2 cloves garlic, minced 1 teaspoon dried basil 1 teaspoon dried rosemary 1 teaspoon dried sage 1 bay leaf Sea salt, to taste 1/2 teaspoon freshly ground black pepper 1/2 cup water 1/2 cup broth, preferably homemade 1 tablespoon soy sauce 1 tablespoon fresh parsley leaves, roughly chopped

Directions

Press the "Sauté" button to heat up your Instant Pot. Once hot, melt the butter and sauté the mushrooms and garlic until aromatic. Add seasonings, water, and broth. Add garlic, oregano, mushrooms, thyme, basil, bay leaves, veggie broth, and salt and pepper to your instant pot. Secure the lid. Choose "Manual" mode and High pressure; cook for 5 minutes. Once cooking is complete, use a quick pressure release; carefully remove the lid. Arrange your mushrooms on a serving platter and serve with cocktail sticks. Bon appétit!

Party Chicken Drumettes

(Ready in about 15 minutes | Servings 8)

Per serving: 237 Calories; 20.6g Fat; 3.1g Carbs; 10.2g Protein; 1.8g Sugars

Ingredients

2 pounds chicken drumettes 1 stick butter 1 tablespoon coconut aminos Sea salt and ground black pepper, to taste 1/2 teaspoon dried dill weed 1/2 teaspoon dried basil 1 teaspoon hot sauce 1 tablespoon fish sauce 1/2 cup tomato sauce 1/2 cup water

Directions

Add all ingredients to your Instant Pot. Secure the lid. Choose "Poultry" mode and High pressure; cook for 10 minutes. Once cooking is complete, use a natural pressure release; carefully remove the lid. Serve at room temperature and enjoy!

Crave-Worthy Balsamic Baby Carrots

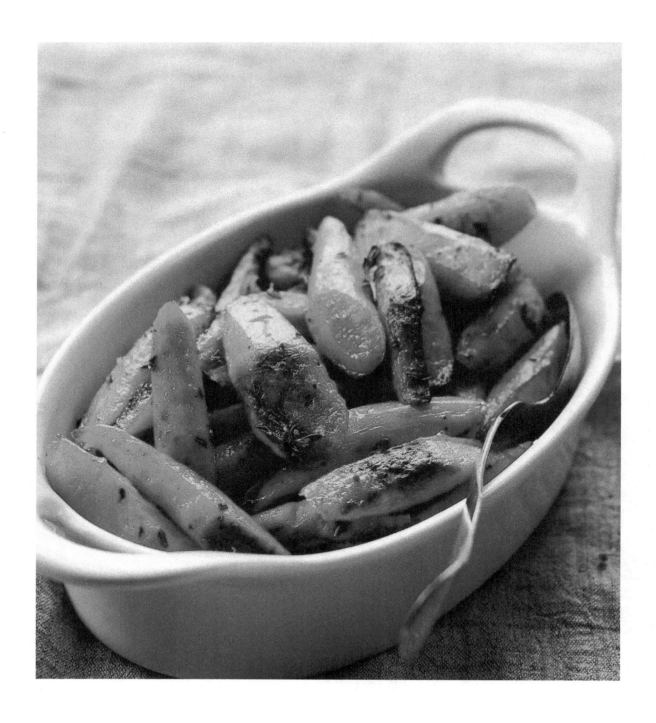

(Ready in about 10 minutes | Servings 8)

Per serving: 94 Calories; 6.1g Fat; 8.9g Carbs; 1.4g Protein; 4.1g Sugars

Ingredients

28 ounces baby carrots 1 cup chicken broth 1/2 cup water 1/2 stick butter 2 tablespoons balsamic vinegar Coarse sea salt, to taste 1/2 teaspoon red pepper flakes, crushed 1/2 teaspoon dried dill weed

Directions

Simply add all of the above ingredients to your Instant Pot. Secure the lid. Choose "Manual" mode and High pressure; cook for 3 minutes. Once cooking is complete, use a quick pressure release; carefully remove the lid. Transfer to a nice serving bowl and serve. Enjoy!

_____

Minty Party Meatballs

(Ready in about 15 minutes | Servings 6)

Per serving: 280 Calories; 20.4g Fat; 3.7g Carbs; 20.6g Protein; 2.5g Sugars

Ingredients

1/2 pound ground pork 1/2 pound ground turkey 2 eggs 1/3 cup almond flour Sea salt and ground black pepper, to taste 2 garlic cloves, minced 1 cup Romano cheese, grated 1 teaspoon dried basil 1/2 teaspoon dried thyme 1/4 cup minced fresh mint, plus more for garnish 1/2 cup beef bone broth 1/2 cup tomatoes, puréed 2 tablespoons scallions

Directions

Thoroughly combine all ingredients, except for broth, tomatoes, and scallions in a mixing bowl. Shape the mixture into 2-inch meatballs and reserve. Add beef bone broth, tomatoes, and scallions to your Instant Pot. Place the meatballs in this sauce. Secure the lid. Choose "Manual" mode and High pressure; cook for 8 minutes. Once cooking is complete, use a quick pressure release; carefully remove the lid. Bon appétit!

Amazing Cauliflower Tots

(Ready in about 25 minutes | Servings 6)

Per serving: 132 Calories; 8.7g Fat; 4.5g Carbs; 9.2g Protein; 1.3g Sugars

Ingredients

1 head of cauliflower, broken into florets 2 eggs, beaten 1 shallot, peeled and chopped 1/2 cup Swiss cheese, grated 1/2 cup Parmesan cheese, grated 2 tablespoons fresh coriander, chopped Sea salt and ground black pepper, to taste

Directions

Start by adding 1 cup of water and a steamer basket to your Instant Pot. Arrange the cauliflower florets in the steamer basket. Secure the lid. Choose "Manual" mode and High pressure; cook for 3 minutes. Once cooking is complete, use a quick pressure release; carefully remove the lid. Mash the cauliflower and add the remaining ingredients. Form the mixture into a tater-tot shape with oiled hands. Place cauliflower tots on a lightly greased baking sheet. Bake in the preheated oven at 390 degrees F approximately 20 minutes; make sure to flip them halfway through the cooking time. Serve at room temperature. Bon appétit!

Gruyère, Rutabaga and Bacon Bites

(Ready in about 10 minutes | Servings 8)

Per serving: 187 Calories; 14.2g Fat; 5.2g Carbs; 9.4g Protein; 3.4g Sugars

Ingredients

1/2 pound rutabaga, grated 4 slices meaty bacon, chopped 7 ounces Gruyère cheese, shredded 3 eggs, beaten 3 tablespoons almond flour 1 teaspoon granulated garlic 1 teaspoon shallot powder Sea salt and ground black pepper, to taste

Directions

Add 1 cup of water and a metal trivet to the Instant Pot. Mix all of the above ingredients until everything is well incorporated. Put the mixture into a silicone pod tray that is previously greased with a nonstick cooking spray. Cover the tray with a sheet of aluminum foil and lower it onto the trivet. Secure the lid. Choose "Manual" mode and Low pressure; cook for 5 minutes. Once cooking is complete, use a quick pressure release; carefully remove the lid. Bon appétit!

Spring Deviled Eggs

(Ready in about 25 minutes | Servings 8)

Per serving: 158 Calories; 12.1g Fat; 2.1g Carbs; 9.5g Protein; 1.2g Sugars

Ingredients

8 eggs Salt and white pepper, to taste 1/4 cup mayonnaise 1/2 can tuna in spring water, drained 2 tablespoons spring onions, finely chopped 1 teaspoon smoked cayenne pepper 1/3 teaspoon fresh or dried dill weed 1 teaspoon Dijon mustard 1 pickled jalapeño, minced

Directions

Place 1 cup of water and a steamer basket in your Instant Pot. Now, arrange the eggs on the steamer basket. Secure the lid. Choose "Manual" mode and Low pressure; cook for 5 minutes. Once cooking is complete, use a quick pressure release; carefully remove the lid. Allow the eggs to cool for 15 minutes. Peel the eggs and slice them into halves. Smash the egg yolks with a fork and add the remaining ingredients. Stir to combine well. Afterwards, stuff the egg whites with tuna mixture. Serve well-chilled and enjoy!

Cheese-Stuffed Cocktail Meatballs

(Ready in about 15 minutes | Servings 8)

Per serving: 277 Calories; 17.4g Fat; 3.1g Carbs; 25.8g Protein; 0.9g Sugars

Ingredients

1 pound ground beef 1/2 cup pork chicharron, crushed 1/2 cup Parmesan cheese, grated 2 eggs, beaten 2 tablespoons fresh scallions, chopped 2 tablespoons fresh cilantro, chopped 1 teaspoon garlic, minced Sea salt, to your liking 1/2 teaspoon ground black pepper 1/2 teaspoon cayenne pepper 1 cup Colby cheese, cubed 2 teaspoons olive oil 1/2 cup chicken broth 1/2 cup BBQ sauce

Directions

In a mixing dish, thoroughly combine ground beef, pork chicharron, Parmesan cheese, eggs, scallions, cilantro, garlic, salt, black pepper, and cayenne pepper; mix until everything is well incorporated. Now, shape the mixture into balls. Press one cheese cube into center of each meatball, sealing it inside. Press the "Sauté" button and heat the olive oil. Sear the meatballs for a couple of minutes or until browned on all sides. Pour in chicken broth and BBQ sauce. Secure the lid. Choose the "Manual" setting and cook for 8 minutes under High pressure. Once cooking is complete, use a quick pressure release; carefully remove the lid. Serve your meatballs with the sauce. Bon appétit!

Bacon Wrapped Cocktail Wieners

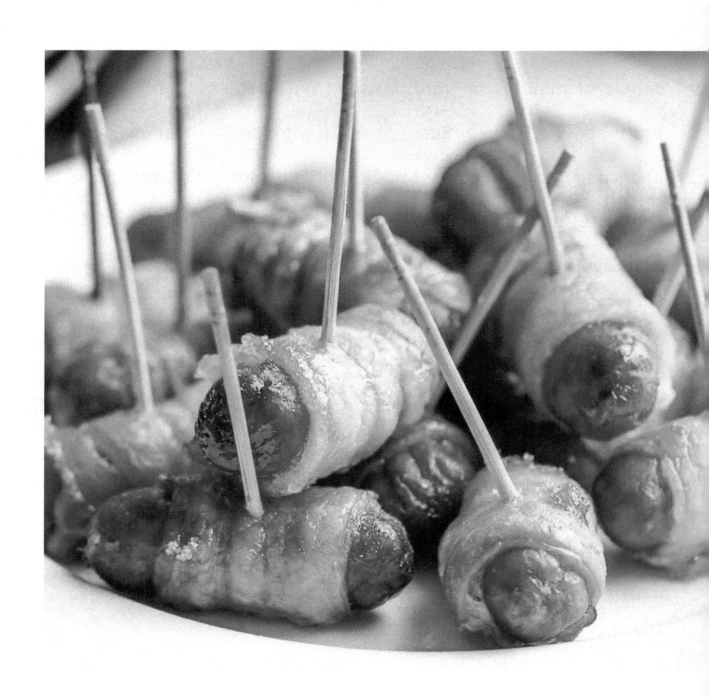

(Ready in about 10 minutes | Servings 10)

Per serving: 257 Calories; 22.7g Fat; 1.4g Carbs; 10.8g Protein; 0.2g Sugars

Ingredients

1 pound cocktail wieners 1/2 pound sliced bacon, cold cut into slices 1/2 cup chicken broth 1/2 cup water 1/4 cup low-carb ketchup 2 tablespoons apple cider vinegar 1 tablespoon onion powder 1 tablespoon ground mustard Salt and pepper to taste

Directions

Wrap each cocktail wiener with a slice of bacon; secure with a toothpick. Then, place one layer of bacon wrapped cocktail wieners in the bottom of the Instant Pot. Repeat layering until you run out of the cocktail wieners. In a mixing bowl, thoroughly combine the remaining ingredients. Pour this mixture over the bacon wrapped cocktail wieners. Secure the lid. Choose "Manual" mode and Low pressure; cook for 3 minutes. Once cooking is complete, use a natural pressure release; carefully remove the lid. Enjoy!

Creole Egg and Pancetta Balls

(Ready in about 25 minutes | Servings 6)

Per serving: 236 Calories; 18.6g Fat; 3.1g Carbs; 13.4g Protein; 1.7g Sugars

Ingredients

6 eggs 1 teaspoon Creole seasonings 1/4 cup mayonnaise 1/4 cup cream cheese 1/3 cup Cheddar cheese, grated Sea salt and ground black pepper, to taste 4 slices pancetta, chopped

Directions

Place 1 cup of water and a steamer basket in your Instant Pot. Now, arrange the eggs on the steamer basket. Secure the lid. Choose "Manual" mode and Low pressure; cook for 5 minutes. Once cooking is complete, use a quick pressure release; carefully remove the lid. Allow the eggs to cool for 15 minutes; then, chop the eggs and add the remaining ingredients; mix to combine well.

Shape the mixture into balls. Serve well-chilled. Keep in the refrigerator up to 4 days.

Chicken Salad Skewers

(Ready in about 10 minutes | Servings 4)

Per serving: 287 Calories; 18.2g Fat; 5.6g Carbs; 24.6g Protein; 2.8g Sugars

Ingredients

1 pound chicken breast halves, boneless and skinless Celery salt and ground black pepper, to taste 1/2 teaspoon Sriracha 1 red onion, cut into wedges 1 cup cherry tomatoes, halved 1 zucchini, cut into thick slices 1/4 cup olives, pitted 2 tablespoons olive oil 1 tablespoon lemon juice, freshly squeezed

Directions

Add 1 cup of water and a metal trivet to the Instant Pot. Arrange the chicken on the metal trivet. Secure the lid. Choose "Poultry" mode and High pressure. Cook the chicken for 5 minutes. Once cooking is complete, use a natural pressure release; carefully remove the lid. Slice the chicken into cubes. Sprinkle chicken cubes with salt, pepper, and Sriracha. Thread chicken cubes, onion, cherry tomatoes, zucchini, and olives onto bamboo skewers. Drizzle olive oil and lemon juice over skewers and serve.

Queso Fundido Dip

(Ready in about 15 minutes | Servings 10)

Per serving: 232 Calories; 19.1g Fat; 2.9g Carbs; 12.1g Protein; 1.5g Sugars

Ingredients

1 pound chorizo sausage, chopped 1/2 cup water 1/2 cup tomato salsa 1 cup cream cheese 1 red onion, chopped 1/4 teaspoon ground black pepper 1/2 teaspoon cayenne pepper 1 teaspoon Mexican oregano 1 teaspoon coriander 1 cup Cotija cheese

Directions

Stir sausage, water, tomato salsa, cream cheese, red onion, black pepper, cayenne pepper, oregano, and coriander into your Instant Pot. Secure the lid. Choose "Manual" mode and High pressure; cook for 6 minutes. Once cooking is complete, use a natural pressure release; carefully remove the lid. Add Cotija cheese and press the "Sauté" button. Stir until everything is heated through.

Enjoy!

Two-Cheese Artichoke Dip

(Ready in about 15 minutes | Servings 10)

Per serving: 204 Calories; 15.4g Fat; 5.6g Carbs; 11.5g Protein; 1.3g Sugars

Ingredients

2 medium-sized artichokes, trimmed and cleaned 1 cup Ricotta cheese, softened 2 cups Monterey-jack cheese, shredded 1/2 cup mayonnaise 1/2 cup Greek yogurt 1 garlic clove, minced 2 tablespoons coriander 1/4 cup scallions 1/4 teaspoon ground black pepper, or more to taste 1 teaspoon dried rosemary

Directions

Start by adding 1 cup of water and a steamer basket to the Instant Pot. Place the artichokes in the steamer basket. Secure the lid. Choose "Manual" mode and High pressure; cook for 8 minutes. Once cooking is complete, use a quick pressure release; carefully remove the lid. Coarsely chop your artichokes and add the remaining ingredients. Press the "Sauté" button and let it simmer until everything is heated through. Bon appétit!

Herbed Party Shrimp

(Ready in about 10 minutes | Servings 4)

Per serving: 142 Calories; 7.5g Fat; 0.2g Carbs; 18.3g Protein; 0g Sugars

Ingredients

2 tablespoons olive oil 3/4 pound shrimp, peeled and deveined 1 teaspoon paprika 1/2 teaspoon dried oregano 1/2 teaspoon dried thyme 1/2 teaspoon dried rosemary 1/2 teaspoon dried basil 1/4 teaspoon red pepper flakes 1 teaspoon dried parsley flakes 1 teaspoon onion powder 1 teaspoon garlic powder Coarse sea salt and ground black pepper, to taste 1 cup chicken broth, preferably homemade

Directions

Press the "Sauté" button and heat the olive oil. Once hot, cook your shrimp for 2 to 3 minutes. Sprinkle all seasoning over your shrimp, pour the chicken broth into your Instant Pot, and secure the lid. Choose "Manual" mode and Low pressure; cook for 2 minutes. Once cooking is complete, use a quick pressure release; carefully remove the lid. Arrange shrimp on a serving platter and serve with toothpicks. Bon appétit!

Asparagus with Greek Aioli

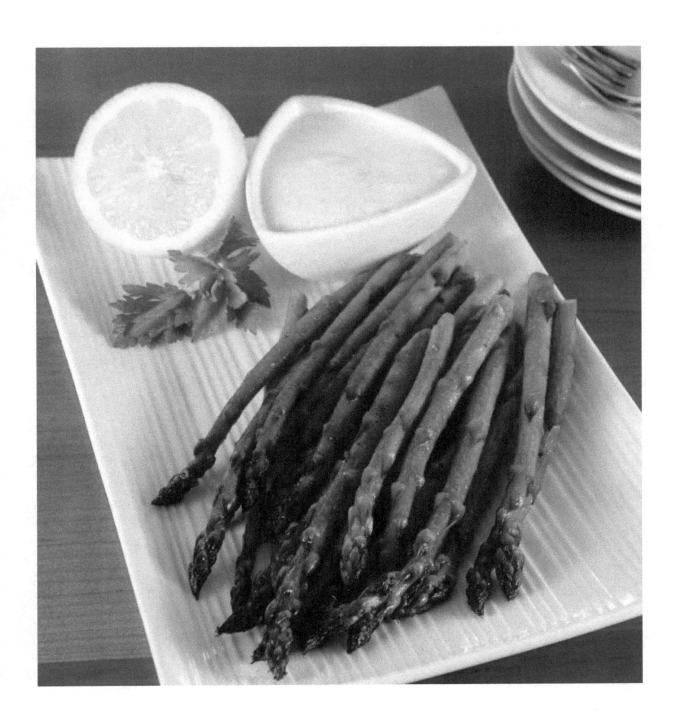

(Ready in about 10 minutes | Servings 6)

Per serving: 194 Calories; 19.2g Fat; 4.5g Carbs; 2.6g Protein; 2.4g Sugars

Ingredients

1 pound asparagus spears Sea salt and ground black pepper, to taste Homemade Aioli Sauce: 1 teaspoon garlic, minced 1 egg yolk 1/2 cup olive oil Sea salt and ground black pepper, to your liking 1/4 cup Greek yogurt 2 teaspoons freshly squeezed lemon juice

Directions

Start by adding 1 cup of water and a steamer basket to the Instant Pot. Place the asparagus in the steamer basket. Secure the lid. Choose "Manual" mode and High pressure; cook for 1 minute. Once cooking is complete, use a quick pressure release; carefully remove the lid. Season your asparagus with salt and pepper; reserve. In a blender or a food processor, mix garlic, egg yolk, and oil until well incorporated. Now, add the salt, ground black pepper, and Greek yogurt. Afterwards, add the lemon juice and mix until your aioli is thickened and emulsified. Serve the reserved asparagus spears with this homemade aioli on the side. Enjoy!

Zingy Zucchini Bites

(Ready in about 10 minutes | Servings 6)

Per serving: 70 Calories; 5.1g Fat; 4.4g Carbs; 3.2g Protein; 0.9g Sugars

Ingredients

2 tablespoons olive oil 1 red chili pepper, chopped 1 pound zucchini, cut into thick slices 1 teaspoon garlic powder 1 cup chicken broth Coarse sea salt and ground black pepper, to taste 1/2 teaspoon paprika 1/2 teaspoon ground coriander

Directions

Press the "Sauté" button and heat the olive oil. Once hot, cook chili pepper for 1 minute. Add the remaining ingredients. Secure the lid. Choose "Manual" mode and Low pressure; cook for 3 minutes. Once cooking is complete, use a quick pressure release; carefully remove the lid. Bon appétit!

Bok Choy Boats with Shrimp Salad

(Ready in about 10 minutes | Servings 8)

Per serving: 124 Calories; 10.6g Fat; 3.1g Carbs; 4.7g Protein; 1.8g Sugars

Ingredients

26 shrimp, cleaned and deveined 2 tablespoons fresh lemon juice 1 cup of water Sea salt and ground black pepper, to taste 2 tomatoes, diced 4 ounces feta cheese, crumbled 1/3 cup olives, pitted and sliced 4 tablespoons olive oil 2 tablespoons apple cider vinegar 8 Bok choy leaves 2 tablespoons fresh basil leaves, snipped 2 tablespoons fresh mint leaves, chopped

Directions

Toss the shrimp and fresh lemon juice in your Instant Pot. Add 1 cup of water. Secure the lid. Choose "Manual" mode and Low pressure; cook for 2 minutes. Once cooking is complete, use a quick pressure release; carefully remove the lid. Season the shrimp with sea salt and ground black pepper, and allow them to cool completely. Toss the shrimp with tomatoes, feta cheese, olives, olive oil, and vinegar. Mound the salad onto each Bok choy leaf and arrange them on a serving platter. Top with basil and mint leaves. Bon appétit!

Stuffed Baby Bell Peppers

(Ready in about 10 minutes | Servings 5)

Per serving: 224 Calories; 17.5g Fat; 9g Carbs; 8.7g Protein; 5.5g Sugars

Ingredients

10 baby bell peppers, seeded and sliced lengthwise 1 tablespoon olive oil 4 ounces cream cheese 4 ounces Monterey-Jack cheese, shredded 1 teaspoon garlic, minced 2 tablespoons scallions, chopped 1/4 teaspoon ground black pepper, or more to taste 1/2 teaspoon cayenne pepper

Directions

Start by adding 1 cup of water and a steamer basket to the Instant Pot. In a mixing bowl, thoroughly combine all ingredients, except for bell peppers. Then, stuff the peppers with cheese mixture. Place the stuffed peppers in the steamer basket. Secure the lid.

Choose "Manual" mode and High pressure; cook for 5 minutes. Once cooking is complete, use a quick pressure release; carefully remove the lid. Serve at room temperature and enjoy!

Barbecue Lil Smokies

(Ready in about 10 minutes | Servings 8)

Per serving: 120 Calories; 4.9g Fat; 1.2g Carbs; 17.5g Protein; 0.6g Sugars

Ingredients

1 ½ pounds beef cocktail wieners 1 cup water 1/4 cup apple cider vinegar 1/2 tablespoon onion powder 1/2 teaspoon ground black pepper 1 teaspoon ground mustard 2 ounces ale

Directions

Simply throw all ingredients into your Instant Pot. Secure the lid. Choose "Manual" mode and High pressure; cook for 2 minutes. Once cooking is complete, use a natural pressure release; carefully remove the lid. Serve with cocktail sticks and enjoy!

Hot Lager Chicken Wings

(Ready in about 15 minutes | Servings 6)

Per serving: 216 Calories; 16.4g Fat; 2.2g Carbs; 12.9g Protein; 0.5g Sugars

Ingredients

2 tablespoons butter, melted 1 pound chicken thighs Coarse sea salt and ground black pepper, to taste 1 teaspoon cayenne pepper 1 teaspoon shallot powder 1 teaspoon garlic powder 1 teaspoon hot sauce 1/2 cup lager 1/2 cup water

Directions

Press the "Sauté" button and melt the butter. Once hot, brown the chicken thighs for 2 minutes per side. Add the remaining ingredients to your Instant Pot. Secure the lid. Choose "Poultry" mode and High pressure; cook for 6 minutes. Once cooking is complete, use a quick pressure release; carefully remove the lid.

Serve at room temperature and enjoy!

Wax Beans with Pancetta

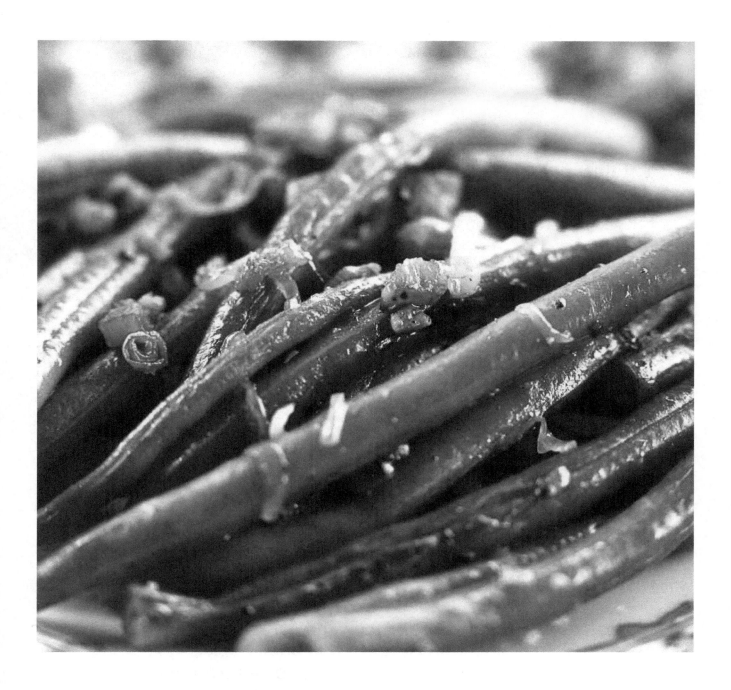

(Ready in about 10 minutes | Servings 6)

Per serving: 194 Calories; 8.7g Fat; 5.8g Carbs; 24.3g Protein; 2.9g Sugars

Ingredients

1 tablespoon peanut oil 1/2 cup shallots, chopped 4 slices pancetta, diced 1 teaspoon roasted garlic paste 1 pound yellow wax beans, cut in half Kosher salt and ground black pepper, to your liking 1 cup water

Directions

Press the "Sauté" button to heat up your Instant Pot. Now, heat the peanut oil and sauté the shallot until softened. Now, add pancetta and continue to cook for a further 3 to 4 minutes; reserve. Add the other ingredients; stir to combine Secure the lid. Choose "Manual" mode and Low pressure; cook for 3 minutes. Once cooking is complete, use a quick pressure release; carefully remove the lid. Serve warm, garnished with the reserved shallots and pancetta. Bon appétit!

Cheesy Cauliflower Bites

(Ready in about 10 minutes | Servings 6)

Per serving: 130 Calories; 9.6g Fat; 5.1g Carbs; 6.9g Protein; 2g Sugars

Ingredients

1 pound cauliflower, broken into florets Sea salt and ground black pepper, to taste 2 tablespoons lemon juice 2 tablespoons extra-virgin olive oil 1 cup Cheddar cheese, preferably freshly grated

Directions

Add 1 cup of water and a steamer basket to your Instant Pot. Now, arrange cauliflower florets on the steamer basket. Secure the lid. Choose "Manual" mode and Low pressure; cook for 3 minutes. Once cooking is complete, use a quick pressure release; carefully remove the lid. Sprinkle salt and pepper over your cauliflower; drizzle with lemon juice and olive oil. Scatter grated cheese over the cauliflower florets. Press the "Sauté" button to heat up your Instant Pot. Let it cook until the cheese is melted or about 5 minutes. Bon appétit!

Sichuan-Style Duck Breast

(Ready in about 2 hours 15 minutes | Servings 4)

Per serving: 256 Calories; 13.7g Fat; 1g Carbs; 29.1g Protein; 0g Sugars

Ingredients 1 pound duck breast, boneless, skinless and cut into 4 pieces 1/2 teaspoon coarse sea salt 1/4 teaspoon Sichuan peppercorn powder 1/2 teaspoon cayenne pepper 2 garlic cloves, minced 2 tablespoons peanut oil 1/2 cup dry red wine 1 tablespoon sake 1/2 cup chicken broth

Directions

Place all ingredients, except for the broth, in the ceramic dish; place the dish in your refrigerator and let it marinate for 1 to 2 hours. Then, transfer the meat along with its marinade to the Instant Pot. Pour in the chicken broth. Secure the lid. Choose "Manual" mode and High pressure; cook for 10 minutes. Once cooking is complete, use a quick pressure release; carefully remove the lid.   Serve warm and enjoy!

.

Chia and Blackberry Jam

(Ready in about 10 minutes | Servings 12)

Per serving: 38 Calories; 1.1g Fat; 8.2g Carbs; 1.2g Protein; 4.7g Sugars

Ingredients

10 ounces fresh blackberries, rinsed 1/2 cup Swerve, powdered 3 teaspoons chia seeds 1/2 cup water

Directions

Add blackberries to your Instant Pot. Sprinkle with Swerve and chia seeds. Pour in 1/2 cup of water. Secure the lid. Choose "Manual" mode and High pressure; cook for 2 minutes. Once cooking is complete, use a natural pressure release; carefully remove the lid. Process the mixture with an immersion blender. Store your jam in a mason jar or serve immediately. Bon appétit!

Japanese-Style Savory Custard

(Ready in about 10 minutes | Servings 4)

Per serving: 206 Calories; 15.3g Fat; 5.5g Carbs; 11.1g Protein; 2.2g Sugars

Ingredients

4 eggs 3/4 cup dashi, cold 1/4 sour cream 2 teaspoons light soy sauce 1 tablespoon sesame oil 1 tablespoon mirin 1/2 yellow onion, minced 2 garlic cloves, minced Salt and pepper, to taste 1/2 cup scallions, chopped

Directions

Prepare the Instant Pot by adding 1 ½ cups of water and a metal rack to its bottom. Whisk the eggs, dashi, sour cream, soy sauce, sesame oil, and mirin in a mixing bowl. Now, strain this mixture over a fine mesh strainer into a baking dish. Add the onions, garlic, salt, and pepper; stir to combine well. Lower the cooking dish onto the rack. Secure the lid. Choose "Steam" mode and High pressure; cook for 6 minutes. Once cooking is complete, use a natural pressure release; carefully remove the lid. Serve garnished with chopped scallions. Enjoy!

Creamy Breakfast "Cereals"

(Ready in about 15 minutes | Servings 4)

Per serving: 185 Calories; 14.4g Fat; 9.2g Carbs; 5.9g Protein; 6.8g Sugars

Ingredients

1/4 coconut flour 1/4 cup almond flour 1 tablespoon flaxseed meal 1/4 teaspoon kosher salt 1/2 cup milk 1/2 cup water 2 eggs, beaten 1/4 stick butter 4 tablespoons Swerve, granulated 2 tablespoons double cream 2 ounces raspberries 1 ounce blueberries

Directions

Add all ingredients to the Instant Pot. Secure the lid. Choose "Manual" mode and High pressure; cook for 5 minutes. Once cooking is complete, use a quick pressure release; carefully remove the lid. Serve garnished with some extra berries if desired.

Enjoy!

_____

Spicy Mushroom Hot Pot

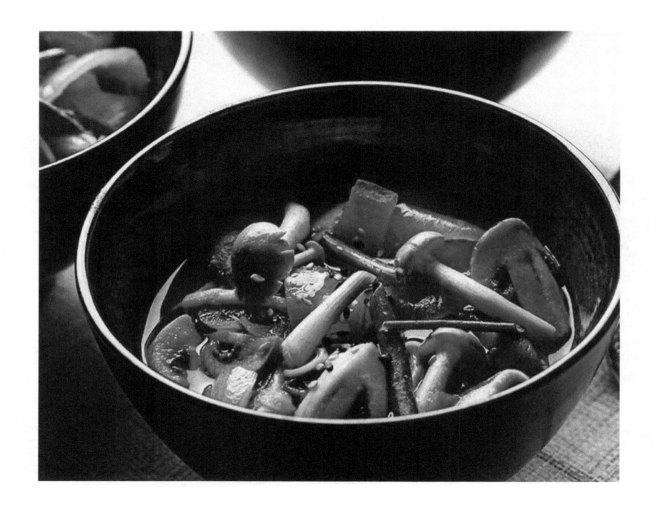

(Ready in about 10 minutes | Servings 4)

Per serving: 195 Calories; 14.3g Fat; 6.8g Carbs; 11.7g Protein; 3.5g Sugars

Ingredients

1 tablespoon olive oil 1 pound white mushrooms, thinly sliced 1/2 onion, chopped 1 cup water Sea salt and ground black pepper, to taste 1 bay leaf 1 cup Colby cheese, shredded

Directions

Press the "Sauté" button to heat up the Instant Pot. Now, heat the oil and cook the mushrooms with onions until softened and fragrant. Add the water, salt, black pepper, and bay leaf. Secure the lid. Choose "Manual" mode and High pressure; cook for 5 minutes. Once cooking is complete, use a quick pressure release; carefully remove the lid. Add cheese, cover with the lid and let it sit in the residual heat until the cheese is melted. Serve warm.

Lobster and Cheese Dip

(Ready in about 20 minutes | Servings 10)

Per serving: 291 Calories; 20.7g Fat; 4.9g Carbs; 21.2g Protein; 3.2g Sugars

Ingredients

2 tablespoons butter 1 onion, chopped 1 celery, chopped 2 garlic cloves, minced 2 tomatoes, puréed 1 cup chicken broth 1 teaspoon Old Bay seasoning Salt and ground black pepper, to taste 1/2 teaspoon paprika 30 ounces frozen lobster 2 cups cream cheese 1 cup Cheddar cheese, shredded

Directions

Press the "Sauté" button to heat up the Instant Pot. Now, melt the butter and sauté the onion and celery until softened. Then, add garlic and continue to cook an additional minute or until aromatic. Add tomatoes, chicken broth, spices, lobster and cream cheese.

Secure the lid. Choose "Manual" mode and Low pressure; cook for 12 minutes. Once cooking is complete, use a quick pressure release; carefully remove the lid. Using an immersion blender, puree the mixture to your desired consistency. Return the mixture to the Instant Pot. Press the "Sauté" button and add Cheddar cheese. Let it simmer until everything is melted and incorporated. Bon appétit!

Cauliflower Breakfast Cups

(Ready in about 15 minutes | Servings 6)

Per serving: 335 Calories; 25.9g Fat; 5.8g Carbs; 19.8g Protein; 2.6g Sugars

Ingredients

1/2 pound cauliflower, riced Sea salt and ground black pepper, to taste 1/2 teaspoon cayenne pepper 1/2 teaspoon dried dill weed 1/2 teaspoon dried basil 1/4 teaspoon dried oregano 2 tablespoons olive oil 2 garlic cloves, minced 1/2 cup scallions, chopped 1 cup Romano cheese, preferably freshly grated Salt and ground black pepper, to taste 7 eggs, beaten 1/2 cup Cotija cheese, grated

Directions

Start by adding 1 ½ cups of water and a metal rack to the bottom of the Instant Pot. Spritz each muffin cup with a nonstick cooking spray. Mix the ingredients until everything is well incorporated.

Now, spoon the mixture into lightly greased muffin cups. Lower the cups onto the rack in the Instant Pot. Secure the lid. Choose "Manual" mode and High pressure; cook for 10 minutes. Once cooking is complete, use a natural pressure release; carefully remove the lid. Bon appétit!

Goat Cheese and Cauliflower Pancake

(Ready in about 35 minutes | Servings 4)

Per serving: 198 Calories; 15.2g Fat; 4.9g Carbs; 11.2g Protein; 1.9g Sugars

Ingredients

3/4 pound cauliflower, riced 4 eggs, beaten 1/2 cup goat cheese, crumbled 1/2 teaspoon onion powder 1 teaspoon garlic powder Sea salt and white pepper, to taste 2 tablespoons butter, melted

Directions

Simply combine all ingredients in a mixing bowl. Now, spritz the bottom and sides of your Instant Pot with a nonstick cooking spray. Pour the batter into the Instant Pot. Secure the lid. Choose "Bean/Chili" mode and Low pressure; cook for 30 minutes. Once cooking is complete, use a natural pressure release; carefully remove the lid. Serve with some extra butter or cream cheese if desired. Bon appétit!

Dad's Chorizo Dip

(Ready in about 15 minutes | Servings 12)

Per serving: 210 Calories; 16.6g Fat; 3.8g Carbs; 11g Protein; 1.5g Sugars

Ingredients

1 tablespoon olive oil 3/4 pound Chorizo, casings removed and crumbled 1 onion, peeled and chopped 15 ounces Ricotta cheese 1/2 teaspoon ground black pepper 2 tablespoons fresh parsley 2 tablespoons fresh chives, chopped

Directions

Press the "Sauté" button to heat up the Instant Pot. Now, heat the oil and brown Chorizo sausage for 2 to 3 minutes. Add the onion, cheese and black pepper to the Instant Pot. Secure the lid. Choose "Manual" mode and High pressure; cook for 10 minutes. Once cooking is complete, use a quick pressure release; carefully remove the lid. Garnish with fresh parsley and chives. Bon appétit!

Favorite Lettuce Wraps

(Ready in about 15 minutes | Servings 6)

Per serving: 301 Calories; 22.1g Fat; 6.2g Carbs; 19.5g Protein; 2.5g Sugars

Ingredients

2 chicken breasts 1 cup chicken stock 2 garlic cloves, minced 1/2 teaspoon black pepper 1 cup green onions, chopped 1 bell pepper, seeded and chopped 1 red chili pepper, seeded and chopped 1 cup cream cheese 1/2 cup mayonnaise 1 teaspoon yellow mustard Sea salt, to taste 1 head of lettuce

Directions

Add chicken breasts, stock, garlic, and black pepper to your Instant Pot. Secure the lid. Choose "Poultry" mode and High pressure; cook for 10 minutes. Once cooking is complete, use a quick pressure release; carefully remove the lid. Then, shred the chicken and divide it between lettuce leaves. Divide the remaining ingredients between lettuce leaves and serve immediately. Bon appétit!

Tacos with Pulled Pork and Pico de Gallo

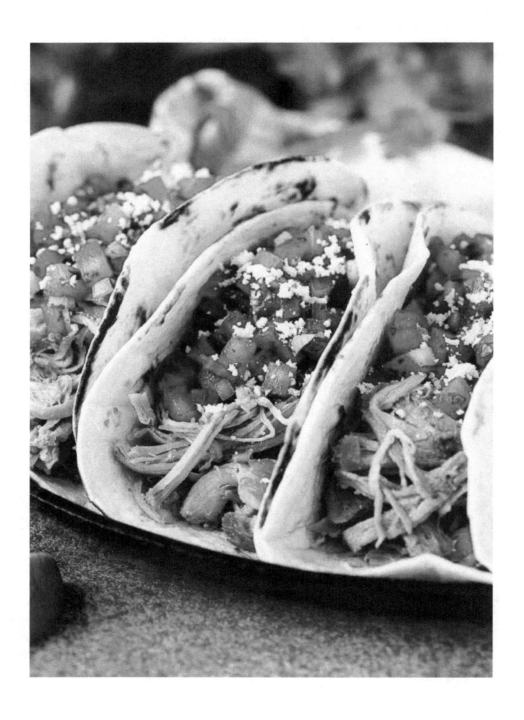

(Ready in about 55 minutes | Servings 4)

Per serving: 429 Calories; 26.7g Fat; 4.4g Carbs; 41g Protein; 2.3g Sugars

Ingredients

1 tablespoon lard, at room temperature 1 pound pork shoulder 1 cup broth, preferably homemade Salt and black pepper, to taste 1/2 teaspoon cayenne pepper 1/2 pound sharp Cheddar cheese, shredded 1 cup Pico de Gallo

Directions

Press the "Sauté" button to heat up the Instant Pot. Melt the lard and sear the pork for 5 minutes, turning occasionally. Use the broth to deglaze the pan. Season with salt, black pepper, and cayenne pepper. Secure the lid. Choose the "Manual" setting and cook for 50 minutes at High pressure. Once cooking is complete, use a natural pressure release; carefully remove the lid. Shred the prepared pork and reserve. Place cheese in a large pile in a preheated pan. When the cheese is bubbling, top it with the meat. Add Pico de Gallo. Afterward, fold over and place on a serving plate. Enjoy!

Egg Salad "Sandwich"

(Ready in about 25 minutes | Servings 4)

Per serving: 406 Calories; 37g Fat; 7.3g Carbs; 11.6g Protein; 4.2g Sugars

Ingredients

6 eggs 1/2 cup tablespoons mayonnaise 1 teaspoon Dijon mustard 1/2 cup cream cheese 1 cup baby spinach Salt and ground black pepper, to taste 2 red bell peppers, sliced into halves 2 green bell pepper, sliced into halves

Directions

Place 1 cup of water and a steamer basket in your Instant Pot. Next, place the eggs in the steamer basket. Secure the lid. Choose "Manual" mode and Low pressure; cook for 5 minutes. Once cooking is complete, use a quick pressure release; carefully remove the lid. Allow the eggs to cool for 15 minutes. Chop the eggs and combine them with mayonnaise, Dijon mustard, cheese, and baby spinach. Season with salt and pepper. Divide the mixture between four bell pepper "sandwiches". Serve well chilled and enjoy!